SAFETY

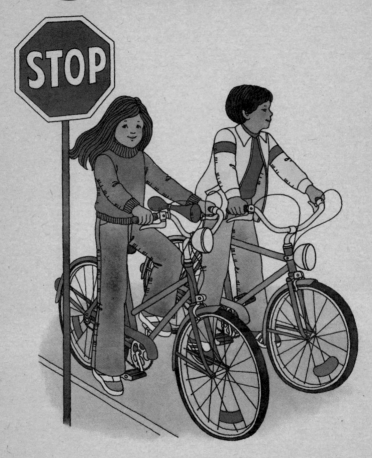

Troll Associates

SAFETY

by Laurence Santrey

Illustrated by Ethel Gold

Troll Associates

Library of Congress Cataloging in Publication Data

Santrey, Laurence.
  Safety.

  Summary: Discusses safety rules to observe at home
and in various situations outdoors.
    1. Safety education—Juvenile literature. [1. Safety]
I. Gold, Ethel, ill. II. Title.
HV675.5.S26   1984   613.6   84-2700
ISBN 0-8167-0230-6 (lib. bdg.)
ISBN 0-8167-0231-4 (pbk.)

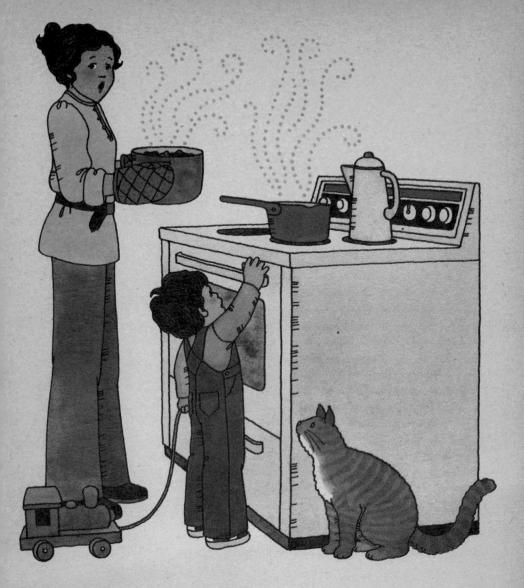

When you were very young, you may
have gone near a stove where someone was
cooking. If you did, an adult probably cried,
"Watch out! It's hot!" Then they may have
picked you up and moved you out of danger.

Now, of course, you know better than to touch a hot stove. You know other rules of safety, too. You know how to cross the street safely and how to ride a bicycle with care. And perhaps you know how to work safely with tools. Practicing safety is important in the home, out-of-doors, in the water—everywhere. Observing safety rules helps to avoid danger and to prevent accidents and injuries.

The key to safety is common sense. Is it common sense to stick your hand inside a beehive? Of course not! The risk of getting stung by a swarm of angry bees is too great. Should you stand on a pile of books to reach a high shelf? Common sense tells you that the risk of falling is too great—so it's better to use a sturdy step stool.

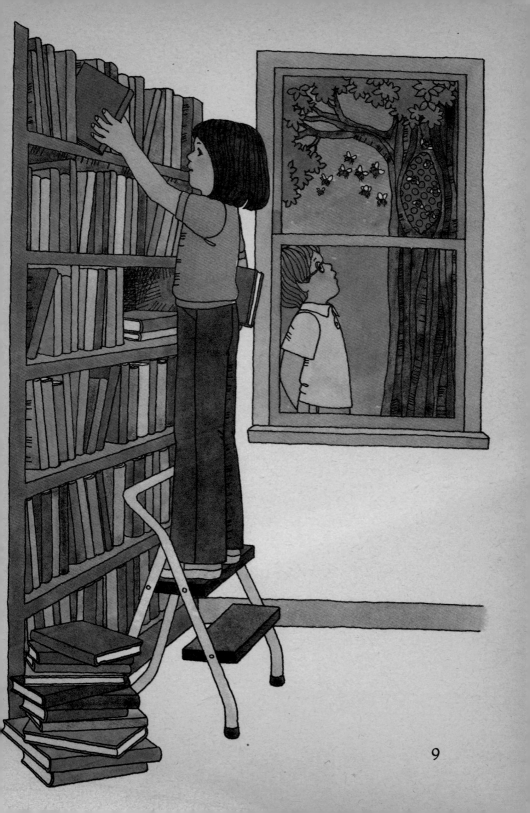

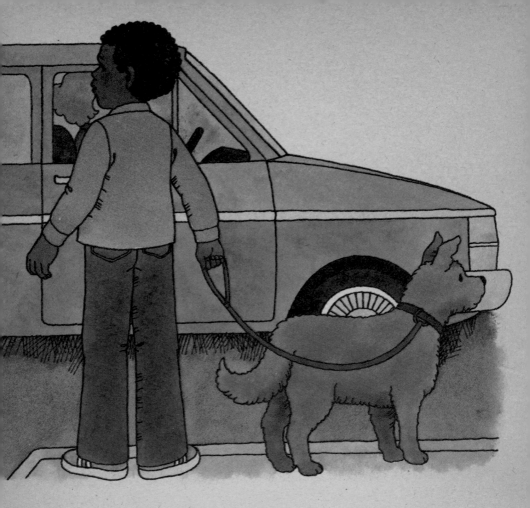

When people aren't alert, they increase
their chances of having an accident. The first
common-sense rule of safety, then, is to be
alert. That's why careful people don't cross
the street with their eyes closed! Instead,
they look both ways before crossing. And
they try to be aware of everything that's
going on all around them.

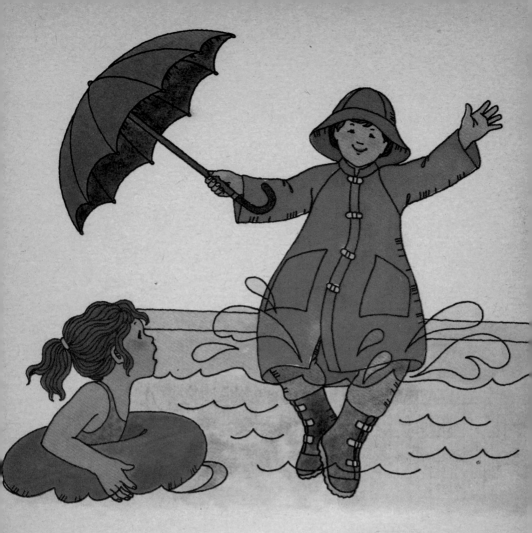

The next common-sense rule of safety is to be properly dressed for whatever you're going to do. It wouldn't make much sense to wear a raincoat and boots in a swimming pool. Not only would they make it impossible for you to swim—they would also look very silly!

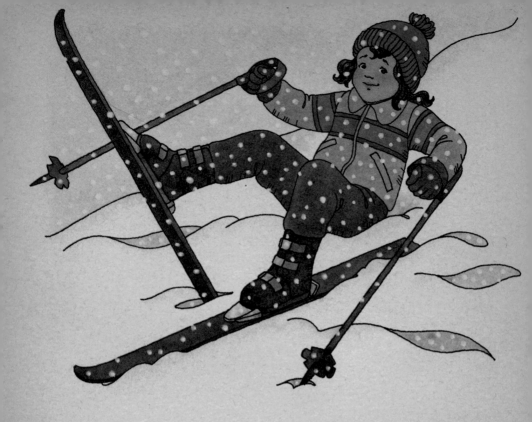

The third rule is to avoid being overconfident or impatient. Unless you're looking for broken bones and bruises, don't try to ski down a steep mountainside the first time you wear a pair of skis!

A good place to begin reviewing the rules of safety is right at home. Lots of accidents can happen in the home. One reason is that people spend so much time at home. Another reason is that there are many potential dangers in a house or an apartment.

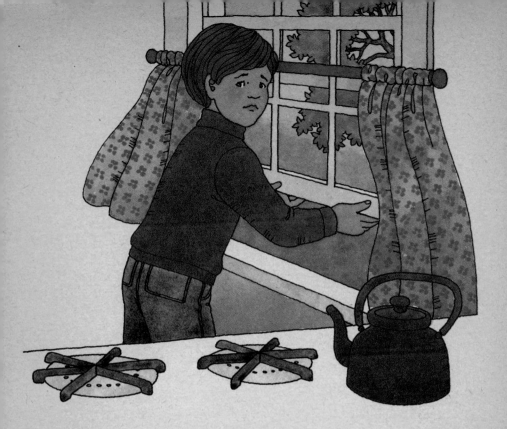

The kitchen is a good place to start. In many homes, the fuel used in the kitchen is gas. Utility companies add a special smell to gas as a safety measure. If there is a gas leak, the smell warns everyone. The first thing to do is open a window. Be sure you do not operate any electrical switches, because even the smallest electrical spark might explode the gas. Leave the area, and call the gas company. They will send someone to repair the leak.

Now, suppose one Saturday afternoon you decide to make some hamburgers for lunch. Everything is going well, until suddenly the grease in the skillet catches fire! What should you do? The first thing to do is smother the fire by putting the lid on the skillet or by pouring baking soda on the burning grease. Never throw water on a grease fire. Water will splatter the hot grease, spreading the fire and burning you.

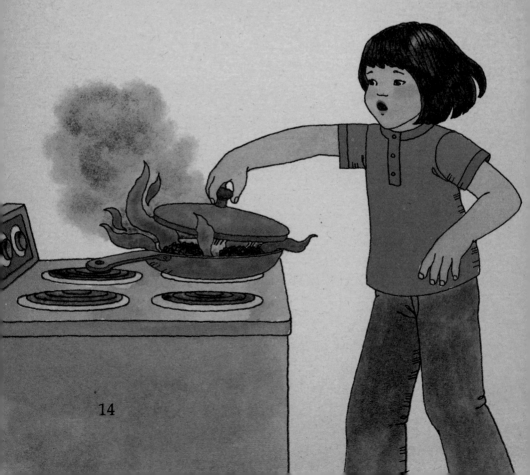

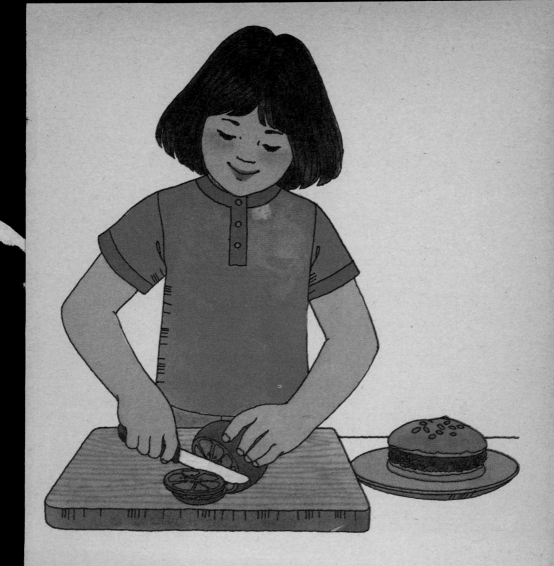

After the grease fire is out, you can finish making your lunch. A nice slice of tomato might taste good on that hamburger. But be careful—knives are sharp. Always cut away from you—not toward you—and be sure that your fingers are clear of the knife blade.

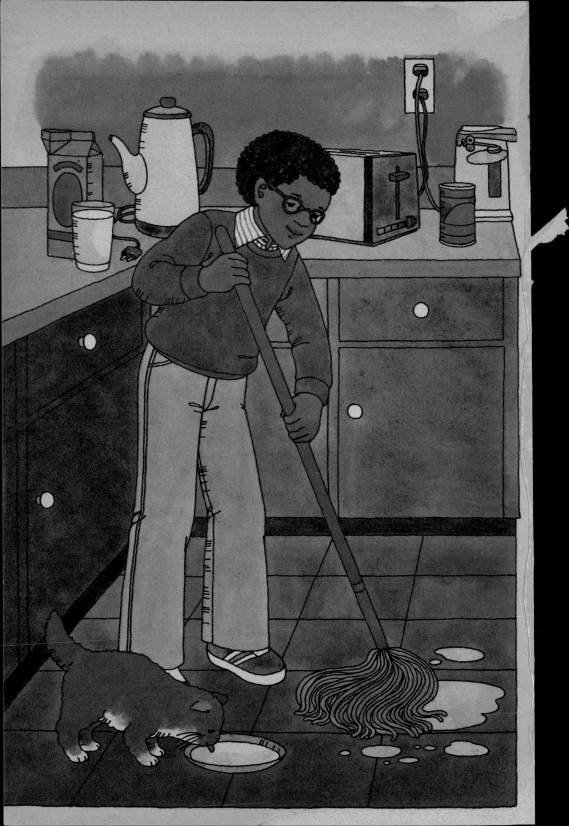

If you should happen to spill some milk, be sure to mop it up—the kitchen floor should always be kept clean and dry, so nobody will slip. Any kitchen equipment that is not being used should be safely out of the way. And, of course, special care should always be taken with electrical appliances.

Toasters and other home appliances such as radios, TV sets, hair dryers, and irons carry enough electrical current to injure or even kill a person. But they are safe when used correctly. To avoid electrical shock, never touch an electrical appliance or switch when any part of your body is in contact with water. Water and other liquids can carry electricity just as well as metal wires do. And so can your body! So be particularly careful around electrical appliances, switches, and outlets.

Opportunities for practicing safety exist all over the house. In the laundry room or bathroom, use common sense when using soaps, detergents, and cleaning liquids. And for safety's sake, keep all medicines out of the reach of children. Never take medicine without adult supervision, and never take anyone else's medicine.

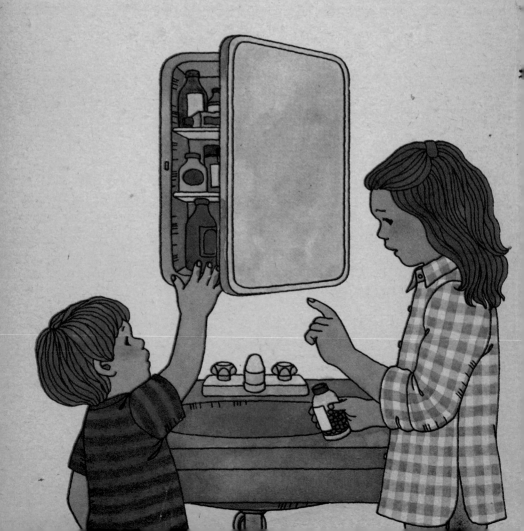

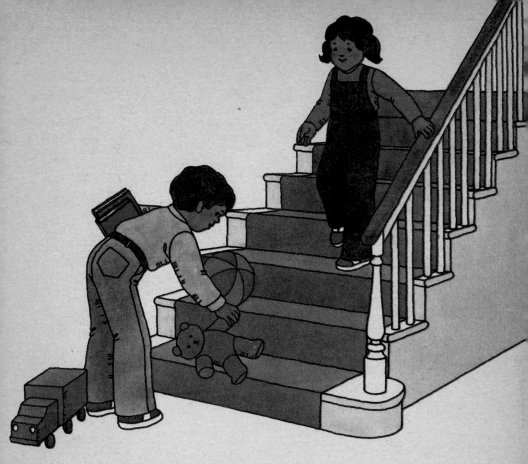

Other safety dos and don'ts to remember include the following: *Do* be careful going up and down the stairs. *Don't* leave books or toys on the stairs for people to fall over. *Do* use hammers, saws, pliers, and other tools safely to protect yourself and anyone working with you. *Don't* play with plastic bags of any kind—they're not toys. And if you must carry sharp objects, like scissors, *do* keep the point down.

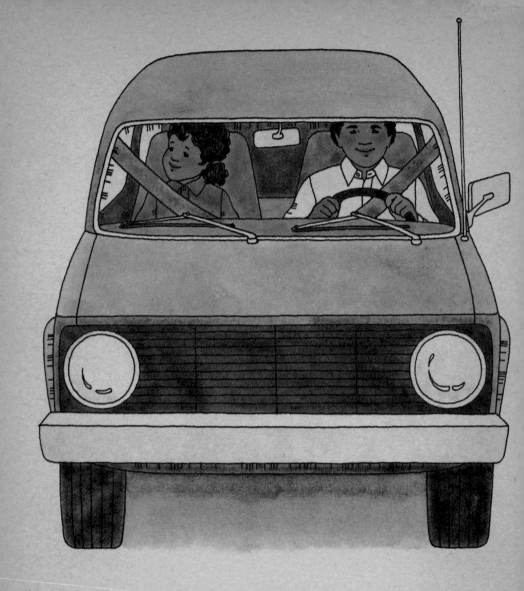

Out-of-doors, there are special safety
rules to follow. Before crossing the street,
look both ways and obey all traffic signals
and signs. In a car or bus, sit still and use seat
belts if they are available. Hanging out of a

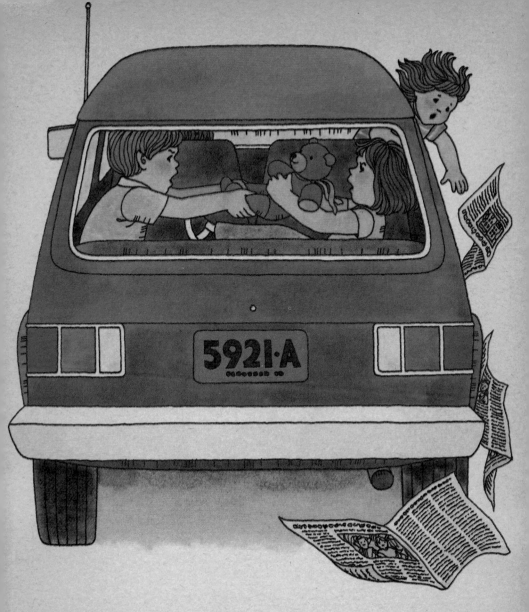

window, jumping up and down, or shoving other passengers are foolish and risky things to do. And anything else that upsets the driver can threaten the safety of everyone.

When riding a bicycle, be sure your bike is safe. Your brakes should be in good working order, and the tires should be properly inflated. It's also a good idea to have lights, a horn, and reflectors. Many communities have bicycle inspections to make sure that these safety standards are met.

Whenever you ride a bicycle, you should

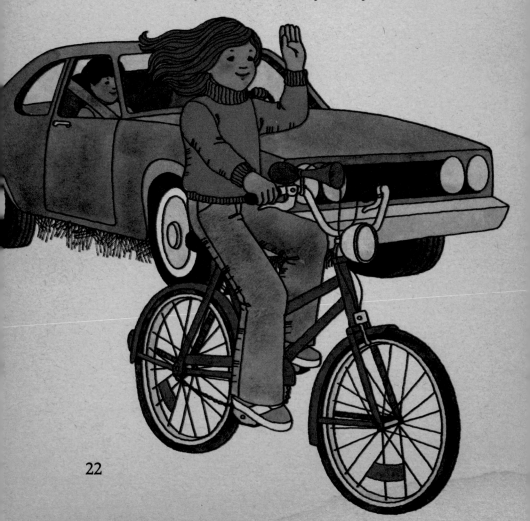

use hand signals to let others know when you are going to turn or stop. Remember to ride on the right side of the street, don't weave in and out of traffic, and never squeeze between two moving vehicles. If you are riding at night, wear light-colored clothing and use your bicycle lights.

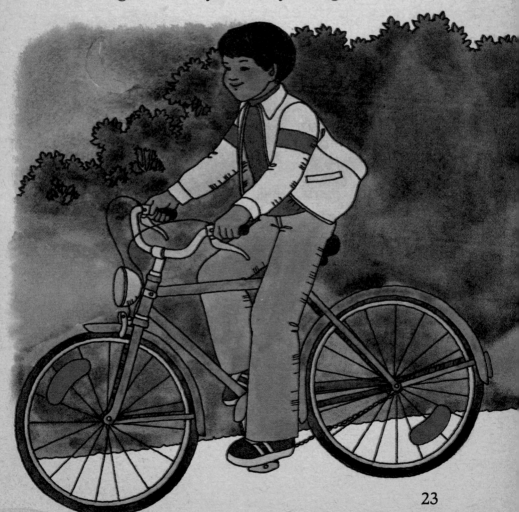

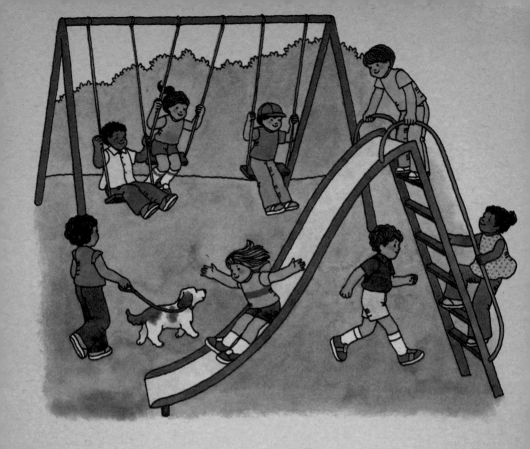

Using playground equipment is lots of fun, particularly when common-sense safety rules are followed. So when one of your friends is using a swing, don't get too close—remember, there are no brakes on a swing! When you want to get off a seesaw, warn the person on the other end. No one likes to come crashing down without a warning. And when you zoom down a slide, make sure nobody is at the bottom.

Nearly everyone loves to go to the beach or jump into a nice cool swimming pool on a hot day. So here are a few safety rules for swimming. First, never swim alone. Even the best swimmers always have at least one buddy with them. And never go swimming unless there is a lifeguard on duty.

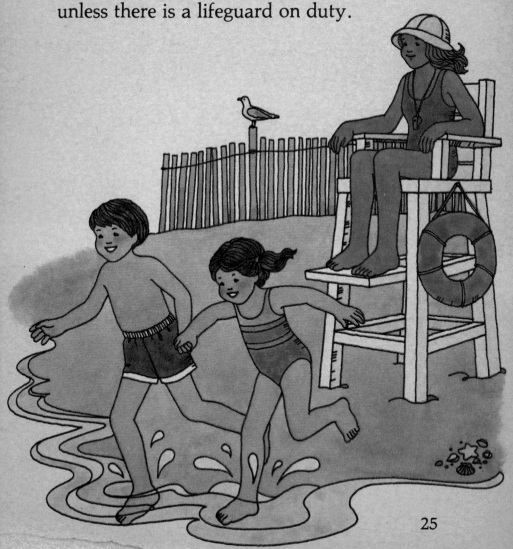

Jumping or diving into unfamiliar water can be a particularly dangerous thing to do, because you won't know the answers to questions like these: Is the water deep enough? Is it too deep? Are there rocks just below the surface? Are there dangerous currents that might drag you out to sea?

Whenever you are swimming in the

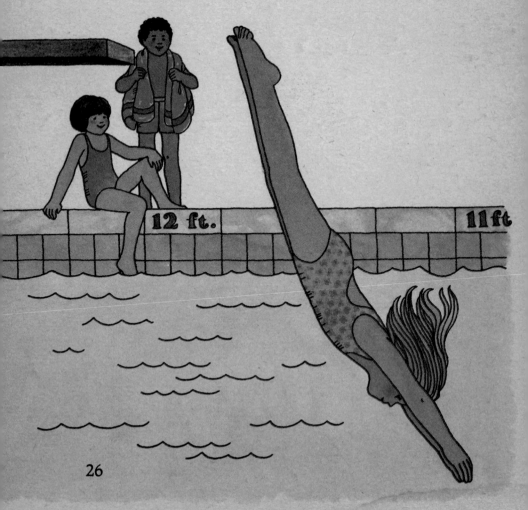

12 ft.   11 ft

ocean, keep in mind that waves can knock a swimmer over, and currents can be strong and unpredictable. If you are carried away from shore by a current, don't panic. Stay afloat and shout for help. If you get a cramp while swimming anywhere, call for help, try to relax, and rub the cramped spot. The most important thing is not to panic.

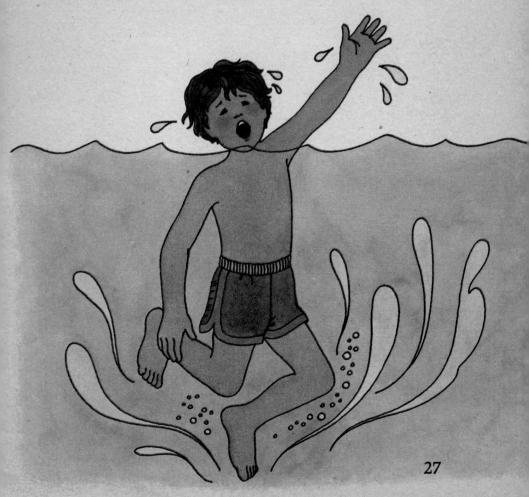

Being a good swimmer is part of boating safety, too. Even though you don't expect to swim to shore from a boat, you should be prepared to. When you are out in a boat, wear an approved life jacket. If you are the operator of the boat, you should know how to handle it, and you should make sure it has a whistle, an anchor, a first-aid kit, signal flares, oars, and a pail for bailing.

Never go out in a boat by yourself. Never stand up in a canoe or rowboat. Never go into waters you are not familiar with. And head for shore at the first sign of a storm. Always make sure an adult knows where you're planning to go and when you'll be back.

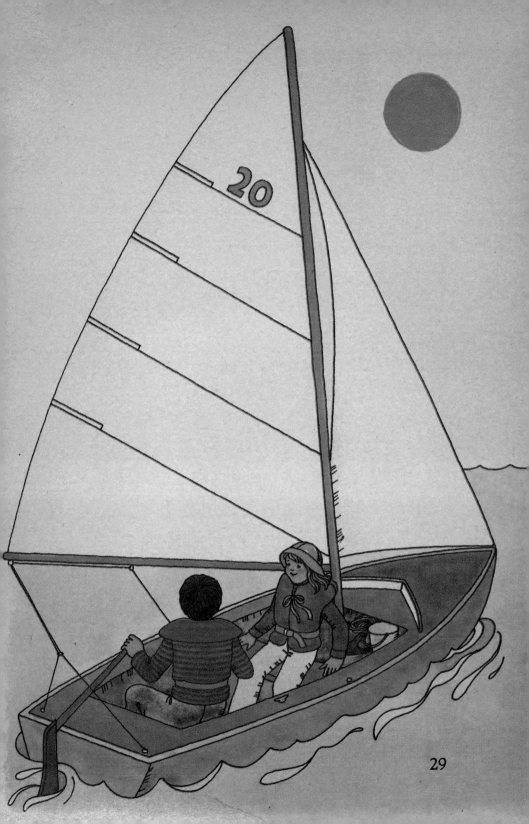

At home or at play, nobody expects to have an accident. But accidents do happen, so it's wise to know what to do in an emergency.

Rule 1: Stay calm and call for adult help, if possible.

Rule 2: Use common sense. You are not a doctor, so don't do anything more than you know how to do.

Rule 3: Take care of the person who is in trouble and don't worry about anything else. Remember that *things* can be replaced, but *people can't.*

Rule 4: Be prepared. There are first-aid courses given by many organizations in the community and school. Try to sign up for one of them.

Finally, as important as it is to know what to do *after* an accident, it is even more important to *avoid* an accident in the first place. And that is what safety is all about!